Anne Cossé

Embrace Menopause

Natural Relief

With Acupressure

Onze Heures Huit

*May this book accompany you during "the Change",
and perhaps make you take advantage of the benefits of
acupressure in other areas of your health and wellbeing.*

Anne Cossé
Certified Acupressure Therapist

Table of Content

Module 1:

Understanding Acupressure

What is acupressure?

How does acupressure work?

Is acupressure safe?

Acupressure Vs western medicine

Why is acupressure so appropriate for women?

What is Acupressure?

Acupressure is a **natural therapy** where the therapist uses gentle to firm finger pressure (as well as the fist, elbow or feet) to stimulate the energy flow in the body, strengthen its self-healing capabilities and enable it to fend off illness better.

Acupressure is one of the three main branches of Traditional Chinese Medicine and is similar to acupuncture except that here the therapist applies pressure to specific pressure points in the body with natural means rather than needles.
Acupressure is often confused with massage, which is quite simplistic by comparison.

The origins of acupressure are as ancient as the instinctive impulse to hold your forehead or temples when you have a headache. Everyone at one time or another has used his/her hands to hold tense or painful places on the body.

More than 5,000 years ago, the Chinese discovered that by pressing certain points on the body, the pain in that pressure point could be relieved. They also found this application of pressure to benefit other parts of the body further away from the pain point.

Gradually, they identified several pressure points that not only alleviated pain but also influenced the functioning of certain internal organs.
A growing number of data and scientific studies show why and how acupuncture and acupressure are efficient, and more and more studies explain and validate the efficiency of this natural healing art.

Acupressure helps to:
- Relieve **physical pain**
- Soothe **muscular tension**
- Boost the **immune system**
- Regulate the **mood and emotions**

To know more about the many benefits of acupressure, visit www.acupressurewellness.com

How Does Acupressure Work?

Acupressure follows the 5,000 year old concepts of Traditional Chinese Medicine.

The vital energy

Eastern tradition describes the world in terms of **energy**. Energy is the elementary substance and vital life force. It is also a synonym of "breath". The Qi evokes breath, movement and vital energy. It encompasses two complimentary aspects: the Yin and the Yang. Without energy, there is no life. All living beings have this energy. It goes way beyond simple muscular energy. It encompasses all the energies a body can pull: **physical, mental, physiological and psychological.**

This flow is called Qi or Ch'i in Chinese (as in Qi Gong and Tai Chi Chuan), Ki in Japanese (as in Aikido) and Prana in India. In the West it is referred to by scientists as bio-electricity and as orgone by Dr W. Reich.

According to traditional Chinese medicine, the Qi is always moving. Ancient Chinese doctors observed that the health of every person depends on the **good circulation** of the vital energy in the body, and on its two polarities, the Yin and the Yang.

The meridians

In the same way that blood is transported by veins, vital energy circulates around the body along a network of **subtle paths**: the Meridians.

The Meridians were identified 5,000 years ago in China.
There are **12 main Meridians**. Eleven of these cross a vital organ and are named after it: Lungs, Large Intestine, Stomach, Spleen, Heart, Small Intestine, Bladder, Kidneys, Pericardium, Gall Bladder, Liver. The 12th Meridian, Triple Warmer, does not relate to any organ.
The 12 Meridians partner in 6 pairs of 1 Yin Meridian and 1 Yang Meridian.
Each Meridian continues to operate if the associated organ is removed. This is also true in cases where a limb has been removed. The Chi of the meridians extends to where the limb would naturally end.

At some specific points along the Meridian paths, the Qi is near the skin and thus physically accessible. These points are the famous acupuncture points, or **acupoints** (called tsubos in Japanese). They are the gateways to the Qi, and to the whole energy system. To work on the acupoints, acupuncture uses needles while acupressure uses gentle to firm finger pressure (as well as the fist, elbow or feet, depending on the technique).

Acupoints are particularly sensitive to bio-electricity, and convey it very quickly. That is how modern science proved their existence.
When the Ki does not flow well, some tsubos become too full or too empty, which generates physical and psychological dysfunction.

The 12 main Meridians are linked together by another layer of 8 Extraordinary Channels. This network regulates the Ki between the Meridians, and hence the harmonious interaction between the organs. The Extraordinary Channels do not have their own acupoints, but flow through the points of more than one main Meridian. Some of those "borrowed" points are Master Points: by simply applying enough to pressure to these Master Points, one can regulate the whole Extraordinary Channel to which it belongs.

The Yin and the Yang

Yin and Yang are **the two sides of everything** in the universe. Outsight and insight, hot and cold, day and night, action and rest, hardness and softness, hallow and deep... one cannot exist without the other.
The Chinese symbol of Yin and Yang perfectly shows this opposition/link: the Yin (in black) and the Yang (in white) are distinct, but create one another (circle) and each one carries the germ of the other (small dot of the opposite color).

The Qi, like electricity, can move thanks to 2 opposing poles. Electricity moves between the positive (+) and negative (-) poles. The Qi moves between the Yin and the Yang.

If the Yin and Yang are out of harmony and balance, the Qi does not flow properly (too strong or too weak, for instance).

The 5 Elements

The Ancient Chinese conceived life and the Universe as a constant interaction between the Yin and Yang. They observed these **relationships in nature** and applied them to the **dynamics of the body**.

The 5 elements are the 5 major characteristics that describe this phenomenon: **wood, fire, earth, metal and water**.

Each element is associated with a yin organ, a yang organ, a body tissue, a sense organ, a body fluid, a flavor, an odor, a moment of the day, an activity, a mental ability, an emotion and a voice type.

Example: Wood = liver, gall bladder, ligaments and tendons, eyes, tears, sour, rancid, morning, beginning, planning, control, anger, loud.

Every human being is made up of the five elements, but one predominates.

An indivisible trio: body, mind and emotions

In Chinese medicine, **the body and mind constantly influence each other**. Emotions are ingrained in the body, and physical pain is a condition of the mind.

Our health and harmony depend on the free and regular flowing of vital energy within our body, mind and emotions.

When any stress disrupts this flow, all the spheres of our being are affected. Not only do we yield to fear, anger and sadness, but we are more prone to illnesses. Depression and anxiety may set in. On the contrary, when body and mind are balanced and in harmony with each other, the energy flows freely, we adjust more easily to a range of emotions, and we feel more joy.

Stress-related tension tends to concentrate on the acupoints. Pressure on these points enables the muscle to stretch and relax, freeing the way to the bloodstream. Toxins are released and flushed away. The bloodstream increase enables more oxygen and nutrients to be conveyed to the body and organs. The body becomes more resistant to disease.

Tension and pain find their source in the accumulation and/or the suppression of negative emotions, and in psychological shocks. That is why acupressure is a valuable ally to restore and strengthen our emotional and psychic balance.

Is Acupressure Safe?

Acupressure **does not involve any intake or mechanical manipulation**. It bears no related side effect, and cannot overwhelm or flood your body.
Its operating mode is to strengthen your body's **own** self-healing capabilities.

In China and in Japan, acupressure is an official medicine. As such, millions of treatments are given every day. In the USA, acupressure has been used since the 1970's. In this country alone, an average of one million injuries caused by medical procedures and drugs side effects are reported in one single year.

Acupressure is safe, when applied or taught by a certified therapist.

However, people experiencing serious medical problems should always consult their doctor before using any alternative therapies. Serious medical conditions include life-threatening diseases, stroke or heart attack, arteriosclerosis, illnesses caused by bacteria, cancer, contagious skin diseases, or sexually transmitted diseases.

Acupressure is **not** used to treat open wounds, scar tissue, varicose veins, or areas of inflammation. If you are experiencing any of these problems, **consult your physician**.

Acupressure Vs Western Medicine

In the West, natural therapies are not a substitute to western medicine. It is recommended to inform your doctors about your using acupressure, and why not showing them this book?

However, many clinical trials – carried out in the USA, UK, Norway, Sweden, China, Taiwan, India… -, prove the efficiency of acupressure and acupuncture for many health issues: nausea and vomiting, pain, insomnia, etc. In more and more countries, hospitals and practitioners use acupuncture and acupressure to complement chemical treatments.

In the case of severe diseases (cancer…) and ailments (post-surgery…), acupressure is recommended as an efficient complementary therapy to alleviate pains associated with the condition or with the drug taking or procedure. The most spectacular example would be with cancer patients, to help them bear the strong side effects of chemo and radio therapy.

In some cases, acupressure or acupuncture are even the primary techniques used by doctors. For instance, many midwives and doctors now use acupuncture and acupressure to induce labor, and ease labor-related pain.

Another common ailment that can be treated with acupressure is lower back pain.

Should you or your physicians have any queries about acupressure and acupuncture efficiency, clinical trials and studies' conclusions are available on www.pubmed.gov, a service of the U.S. National Library of Medicine and the National Institutes of Health.

Why Is Acupressure So Appropriate For Women?

Acupressure is particularly suitable for women, so much in its essence (for women, body and mind, physical and psychological/emotional spheres are strongly intertwined), than in its modality: it is a soft, non-invasive technique, received fully-clothed.

General health

Common women ailments include PMS, cramps, mood swings, menstrual cycle disorders, fertility, ovarian cyst, cystitis, hyperthyroidism, endometritis, breast mascosis, pelvic inflammation, bladder and vaginal infections, eating disorders, anemia. Acupressure is an efficient complementary treatment that regulates the female genito-urinary system, and is a powerful tool to balance emotions.

Maternity

Acupressure helps dealing with the changes, risks and specific ailments related to pregnancy, from conception to delivery, and then during the delicate post-partum time.

- **Prenatal:** relax, release stress and tension, balance mood and feelings, strengthen the bond with child, relieve physical symptoms associated with pregnancy, such as bloating, water retention, muscular cramps, pain in the neck, the back, the hips, sciatica, headaches, nausea, blood pressure, bloodstream.
- **Delivery:** induce a late labour, ease the expulsion process, and relieve pain.
- **Postnatal:** strengthen the natural ability of the body to heal after a vaginal or abdominal delivery. Many women suffer from tension in the neck and shoulders, stress and fatigue, postnatal depression, lactation issues, genital disorders. Acupressure treatment after delivery helps decreasing those symptoms naturally.

Menopause

Menopausal symptoms are the visible part of the hormonal storm that rages in the woman's body. Because acupressure works on balancing, it helps calming the tornado, and supports the woman during this period.

Emotional release

For many reasons, including biological, women are in close contact with their emotions, and need to manage and process them regularly. If verbalization is not possible, women can find in acupressure an efficient mean to rebalance their daily life emotional turmoil.

Low spirits, depression, suffering

Statistics all over the world show that amongst people suffering from depression, there are twice as many women as there are men... Furthermore, women are more prone than men to atypical forms of depression, such as bulimia, hypersomnia, and compulsive buying.

Of course, depression can be triggered by hormones (baby blues, menopause, winter...), but the experts agree that hormones do not explain everything. They think that women are not more prone to depression than men, it's just that they express it more. It is true that women consult therapists, and generally express themselves more easily than men, but one has to admit that they also are subjected to heavy pressure and duties. It is a proven fact that stress affects the "hormones of happiness" - melatonin, noradrenalin, serotonin, endorphins - that regulate mood and well-being. Acupressure helps stimulate them, and resist.

Violence & harassment

Violence, be it physical (assault, sexual abuse) or verbal (harassment, humiliation, emotional blackmail), leaves deep scars in the body and the mind. Acupressure, coupled with verbal therapies (psychotherapy), and practiced in a context of trust and compassion, proves a precious help on the long and difficult path to healing.

> Acupressure is a fit answer
> to women's needs

Module 2:

Guidelines to Practicing Self-Acupressure

How do I locate the points?

How do I work on the points?

How much pressure should I apply?

What else should I do?

How Do I locate The Points?

The practical way to locate the acupoints on your body is to use **anatomical landmarks.** That is how practitioners can find the points on their patients' body, even though bodies come in so many forms and shapes!

Anatomical landmarks are mainly the bone indentations and protrusions, but also creases and articulations, muscles joints and cords, and miscellaneous elements such as the navel, the eye brows...

All the points in this book are illustrated with a description of these landmarks, in addition of pictures.

If you need to refer to a chart to locate a point, here is the way to go. Each point is assigned an **identification number** to track its placement along the body. It is made of the meridian name initial, and the sequence order of that point along the meridian. For instance: K3 = 3rd point on the Kidneys meridian), GB41 = 41th point on the Gall Bladder meridian.

This is the standard referencing system used by professional acupressure practitioners and acupuncturists around the world.

You do NOT need to know or remember any of these numbers to practice the self-acupressure techniques in this book. But you might be interested in looking at meridian charts, in which case you can use the identification number given in this book.

Finally, each point has a **name**, which translation from Chinese to English is not always easy (some points bear more than one translation...). The name is related to the point's main benefit or characteristic. It is sometimes clear (like in "Sea of Energy", or "Facial Beauty"), but often times too obscure for the western mind ("Jumping Circle", "Elegant Mansion"). Not very useful, then, but so poetic!

In this book, we focus on the anatomical landmarks.
The meridian identification letters are:

B = Bladder	LI = Large Intestine	SI = Small Intestine
GB = Gall Bladder	Lu = Lungs	Sp = Spleen
H = Heart	Lv = Liver	St = Stomach
K= Kidneys	P = Pericardium	TW = Triple Warmer

How Do I Work The Points?

There are several different techniques, including movement, rhythm and pressure, to work on the acupoints, which make for different acupressure styles. It goes from the softest (just lightly touching the point) to the hardest (deep firm penetration).

The techniques depend on the point location: points sitting on a strong ropy muscle call for firmness, whereas points sitting on fragile areas (e.g.: around the eyes) can take light touch only.

They also depend on the desired effect: pressing with an intermittent, fast beat is stimulating; a slower pressure creates a deeply relaxing effect on the body; tapping generates vibrations and "awakens' the whole meridian.

In this book, we'll use the following easy techniques:

Firm steady pressure is the most common technique. The thumbs are mainly used, but the others fingers, the palms, and the knuckles are often useful to apply stationary pressure.
There are two ways to apply pressure:
- Hold the point without any movement for a few seconds to several minutes at a time.
- A series of short, firm pressures lasting a few seconds, about eight to twelve times.

Firm pressure with rotation: After applying steady, firm pressure directly on the acupoint, massage it with a slow rotating movement. Keep the circular movement small, so that you keep stimulating the right spot. Start with light pressure and gradually build up to a level before pain.

Rubbing uses brisk friction to stimulate the blood and lymph. It is appropriate for larger areas of the body, such as the back. Make a loose fist, and rub the skin lightly with your knuckles.

How Do I Apply Pressure?

Always use the pulp of your finger tips, not the tip itself:

Yes   No

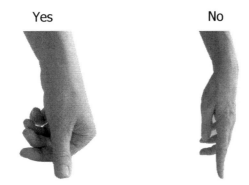

Depending on the point, you can use one or more fingers:

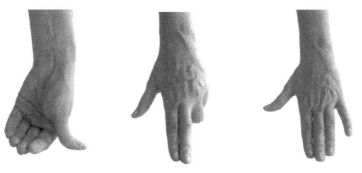

Whatever the technique, there are **3 steps to follow**:
1. Place your finger lightly on the point, as to make a gentle connection.
2. Begin building the pressure gently, at a 90 degree angle from the surface of the skin, and deepen it gradually.
3. Release the pressure slowly, but faster than the build-up.

A golden rule is to **use your body weight** instead of your muscle strength. That way, you do not tire your hands and arms. Whenever anatomically possible, **lean forward** into the point.

To spare your thumb, support it with the other fingers of the same hand, or use paired thumbs.

Tip: If your hand hurts, use tools such as a golf ball or a pencil eraser.

Finally, each acupoint feels differently when you press it. But always remember that **pain is not necessary**! The pressure should be firm enough so that it "hurts good" (in Chinese: "the exquisite pain"). Efficiency is NOT measured by the level of pain you experience. Some acupressure techniques use very light touch, yet they are extremely powerful.

If you feel extreme (or increasing) sensitivity or pain, gradually decrease the pressure until you find a balance between pain and pleasure. After working on the point for a few days, you will discover that the pain will diminish.

What Else Should I Do?

Get prepared

. Wear comfortable clothing
Tight pants, tops, collars, belts, or shoes can obstruct circulation. It is recommended to wear natural fibers that breathe, such as cotton, linen, silk or wool blends. Also, try to keep your fingernails trimmed fairly short to prevent any discomfort or injury to the skin.

. Don't fill your stomach
Digestion takes up to 60% of the body's energy. Wait until at least an hour after eating a light meal and even longer after eating a heavy meal. Avoid iced drinks (especially during the winter months), because extreme cold generally weakens your system and can counteract the benefits of acupressure.

. Avoid alcohol
Alcohol seriously disturbs the energy flow, as well as many vital organs.

Practice in a relaxing environment
Greater benefits are achieved with deep relaxation. Whenever possible, create a comfortable, private environment. Choose a room where you will not be disturbed, and inform your entourage you need to be alone for 15mn.
You can burn essential oils, or light incense, play soft music, light candles, and even stay in the dark, whatever suits you.

Breathe deeply
Concentrate on breathing slowly and deeply while you practice. Deep breathing helps to regulate your metabolism, enhancing the benefits of the exercises and massage. Long and deep breathing brings more oxygen in the body cells, and the organs function better. It helps your body heal itself, and induces relaxation.
When working on a sore or painful acupoint, focus your attention on the painful spot, inhale deeply, and imagine that you are breathing healing energy into the affected area. Do not use a rotation movement. Exhale slowly, letting the healing energy circulate throughout your body. Repeat for three full minutes. It will close the nervous system's pain gates and help the area heal. This breathing technique enhances the healing benefits of all the acupressure exercises in this book.

Practice regularly

For optimal results, and to prevent recurrence, you should practice daily, even after you have obtained relief. If you cannot practice every day, try to treat yourself two or three times a week.

Close the session

Following your routine, give yourself a few minutes to deeply relax on your back with your eyes closed. When you have only a couple of minutes at the end of the routine to relax, you can let yourself relax in a sitting position. First, rub the palms of your hands together briskly to create heat. Close your eyes and immediately place your hands lightly over your face as you breathe deeper than you normally breathe. After a minute, let your hands float into your lap and completely relax for a couple of minutes to discover the benefits.

Having a cup of hot herbal tea is a good idea after an acupressure session along with a period of deep relaxation.

Module 3:

Acupressure Points for Menopause Relief

Control your weight

Dissolve water retention

Balance your mood swings

Lower your anxiety

Calm your irritability

Reduce hot flashes and night sweats

Increase your energy

Sleep better

Strengthen your body's resistance

Reconnect with your libido

CONTROL YOUR WEIGHT

Why Do We Gain Weight During Menopause?

The hormonal imbalance that takes place during pre-menopause and menopause generates a loss of the ability to feel saturation, and a crave for strong taste food (salty, spicy, sweety). Menopausal women, like pregnant women, cannot control easily their eating.

In addition, the emotional and psychological stress that women experience during menopause lowers some of their endorphins levels, which in turn increases cravings.

Finally, the drop in estrogen levels slows down the metabolism. So even if they eat less, menopausal women still gain weight.

Interestingly, at this time, women will find that they tend to put on much of the weight in their abs, not in the rear or thighs, as women tend to do in their younger years. This is when many women generally grow into an 'apple' shape. During this period in your life, it gets harder to equally distribute your body weight. The culprit is known as Androgen, the hormone that is produced in excess during menopause and which causes excess belly fat creation. In addition, declining estrogens and progesterone levels directly encourage the body to store fat desperately.

The good news, however, is that it is possible to stop menopause weight gain if you are prepared to meet the challenge head on and put in some work.

How to Stop Menopausal Weight Gain?

Here are some helpful tips for you.
The 2 Golden Rules:

- **Eat Sensibly**
  Make it a point to eat healthy. A part from the obvious "eat more green vegetables, cut back on carbs and fat", the tips below give you fun ideas to balance your diet.

- **Find New Ways of Exercising**
  It is not about hitting the gym every day; it is about moving it on and enjoying it. For instance, walk as much as possible. You do not need to become an athlete!

20 Fun & Easy Tips to Stop Menopausal Weight Gain:

1. Dance to your favorite music for 15 minutes a day.
2. Park your car a little further and walk. Alight 1 bus station before your usual station. You will discover new streets, shops, etc. Join a walking group if you don't feel confident walking on your own. Now is the time to purchase a pedometer and walk 10.000 steps a day
3. Take the stairs. No lift, no escalator. If you have to take an escalator, climb its stairs.
4. Cut back on sugar, and avoid artificial sweeteners. Do not cut sugar off completely, you need the energy.
5. Spread dry herbs on all your food (parsley, chives, etc).
6. Learn to relax with meditation; stress can lead to more sugar consumption and over eating. If you cannot meditate, buy a guided visualization CD, and just follow the voice. Try this "meditation for dummies", based on acupressure points.
7. Cut back on bread and pasta. Eat organic carbs.
8. Drink eight glasses of water a day. To remember to do so, set the alarm on your phone/PDA/PC. Another trick I find useful is right after going to the toilets, drink as much water as you just released.
9. To eat more fruits, include them in your main dish instead of carbs. Try fusion cuisine recipes, it is fun! Cooked mangoes, apples, and peaches taste great as side dishes.
10. Cut back on coffee and try to drink it black or use skimmed milk.
11. Drink green tea and herbal tea. Pay a visit to your local organic food store, and explore!
12. Replace TV snacks with raw vegetables and fruit.
13. Completely give up sodas of any kind; they contain a lot of sugar or aspartame both to be avoided. Yes, even the "light" and "diet" ones...
14. Enroll in fun dance classes such as aerobic dancing. Guaranteed fun with belly dance and salsa ladies styling!
15. Never forget to eat proteins. If in the evening you have a homemade vegetable soup, add tofu or steamed white meat. Proteins are the bricks our body needs. What triggers hunger is the lack of proteins.
16. Eat 5–6 small meals a day, as opposed to 3 big meals a day.
17. Add omega3s to your diet by eating more sardines or salmon. If you buy these fish in cans, choose the ones in spring water instead of in oil.
18. Take a half hour brisk walk each evening, or morning.
19. Read product labels before buying them to make sure you're eating healthy food.
20. Do NOT starve yourself. You need to energize your body, so don't go on a hunger strike.

To lose weight after menopause takes some work and maybe some lifestyle changes.

Fortunately, **there are many acupoints to use to help in weight management.**

This chapter shows the ones that are appropriate in the context of menopause:
- To **reduce sugar cravings and excessive appetite**
- To **boost the metabolism**

You will find below separate acupoints to stimulate, and at the end of this chapter a full routine to practice every day that also includes acupoints for swelling and water retention.

Abdominal Sorrow

Names: Spleen 16 (Sp16), Abdominal Sorrow

Where: Below the edge of the rib cage, ½ inch from the vertical nipple line.

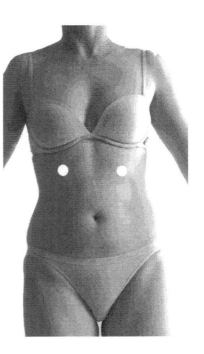

How: Curve your fingers, placing your fingertips in the indentation underneath the edge of the ribs. Press firmly in the indentations for one minute, and breathe slowly.

If you are standing up, press upward and lean your body forward to use your body weight for pressure.

This point is located on the meridian that irrigates the spleen, so it regulates the gastrointestinal system.

Cravings can be triggered by emotional stress. To balance your emotional stress, work that point:

Center of Power

Names: Conception Vessel 12, CV12, Center of Power.

Where: This point is located on the Solar Plexus chakra, hence is name.

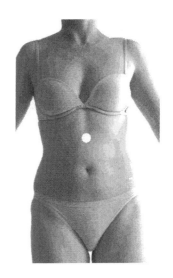

More precisely, it is sitting in the centre of the abdomen, on the midline between the base of the breastbone and the belly button.

How: Standing up, sitting down, or laying on your back, place all the fingertips of both hands along the midline below the breastbone. Press *gradually*, at an upward angle toward the center of your back. You can lean your body forward. Breathe deeply as you hold for one minute.

Caution: In general, it is recommended to work this point for not more than 2 minutes, and not right after a meal. Do not press firmly on this point or rub it briskly or tap it if you have a serious illness.

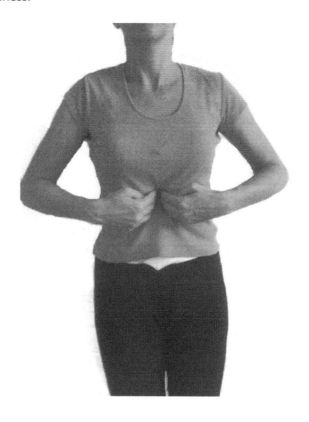

BOOST YOUR METABOLISM

When our metabolism is high, we digest more efficiently, so when we eat the same amount of food, we don't feel hungry shortly after.
An efficient way to stimulate your metabolism is to increase your general energy level.

Key acupoints:

Please see Chapter "Increase your energy" to discover all the points and exercises to boost your vital energy.

Daily exercise

Lie down on your back, with your knees bent and your feet flat on the floor. This routine can be done sitting, although it is less effective.

1. Firmly press CV6 (abdomen):
Place all your fingertips of both hands between the pubic bone and the belly button. Take long deep breaths as you gradually press 1 or 2 inches deep inside the abdomen, and as you apply firm pressure for 1mn.
Caution: Press this point LIGHTLY if you have had a recent abdominal operation, or if you have serious, life-threatening illness (heart disease, cancer, high blood pressure).

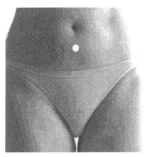

Lightly press Sp9 and Sp6 (inner leg):
With your legs bent and your feet flat on the floor, place your right foot comfortably on your left thigh. Use your right thumb to gently press the right Sp9 point. Use your left thumb to press Sp6. Close your eyes, and breathe deeply for 1mn. Hold the points lightly for another 2 long breaths. Then switch legs.

2. Press K2 and K6 (foot):
Place your foot as in Step 2. Use your right fingertips to press the right K6. Place your left thumb on the right K2. Hold these points for 1mn. Then switch legs. Breathe deeply.

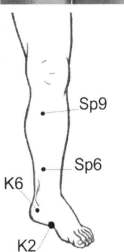

DISSOLVE WATER RETENTION

There are five pressure points on the body that are believed to help with water retention. Working on these points can help you get better quicker.

You do not have to use all of these points. Using just one or two of them whenever you have a free hand can be effective.

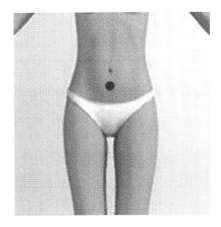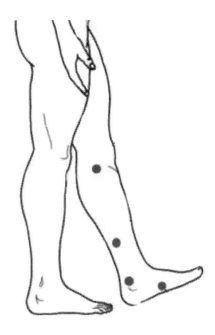

TUMMY POINT:

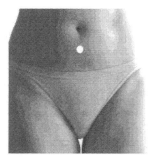

Relieves water retention, chronic diarrhoea, constipation, and gas.

Names:
Conception Vessel 6 (CV6), Sea of Energy, Hara

Where:
Two finger widths directly below the belly button.

How:
You can place your three middle fingers of either hand, on the point area, and press down an inch or two until you reach a firm spot.

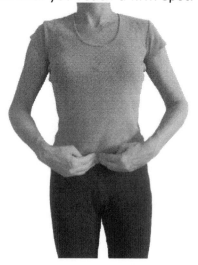

Or, you can use a more relaxed hold and place the palm of one hand gently on your belly, below your belly button, right over the point. You can use one hand, or both, with one hand over the other.

Remember to relax your hands and arms and shoulders. You can hold this while standing (evenly on both feet), sitting (with both feet flat on the ground, back straight), or lying down.

Hold for one or two minutes, while taking slow deep breaths.

UPPER INNER LEG POINT:

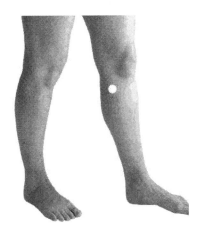

This point is known to relieve water retention but also knee problems, swelling, leg tension, varicose veins, oedema and cramps.

Names:
Spleen 9, Sp9, Shady Side of the Mountain, Yin Ling Quan.

Where:
On the inside of the leg in the depression right below a rounded prominence in the top of the leg bone (tibia).

How:
Place your left thumb on the right leg point and press in the depression, slightly upwards.
Remember to relax your shoulders. Hold for one or two minutes, while taking slow deep breaths.
Switch sides: place your right thumb on the left leg point, press in the depression, slightly upwards, relax your shoulders, old for one or two minutes, while taking slow deep breaths.

LOWER INNER LEG POINT:

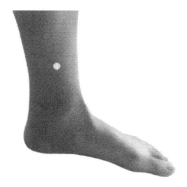

This point is very versatile. It sits where the Spleen, Kidney and Liver meridians intersect and is a very powerful point. It can treat many conditions associated with all three organs. If you have digestive, gynaecological or emotional conditions, just find the point and massage it. It may be tender but do this for two minutes. The tenderness should subside and so should the symptoms.

Names:
Spleen 6, Sp6, San Yin Jiao, Three Yin Intersection.

Where:
This point is located on the inner side of the leg (on the back inner border of the shinbone), four finger widths above the inner anklebone.

How:
Sit down and place your left ankle on your right knee. Place your right hand fingers (except the thumb) on the area above the ankle. That will help you locate the point.

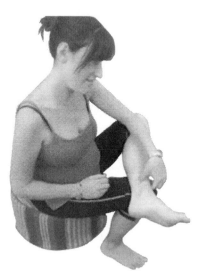

Press with your thumb or knuckle. Increase pressure until you are pressing quite firmly, hold about a minute, and gradually release. Switch legs and work on the right leg point.

Caution: Do not press this point if you are pregnant.

LOWER INNER LEG POINT:

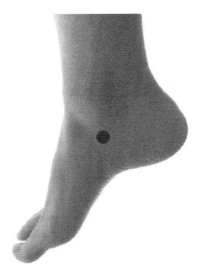

This point is another very versatile acupressure point. I include it in this Weight Loss Program because it relieves water retention and oedema in the legs, especially swollen ankles. In addition it relieves sore throat, swollen, dry, loss of voice, difficulty swallowing, a range of menstrual issues (amenorrhea, dysmenorrhoea, infertility from cold in the uterus, leucorrhoea), genital issues (swelling, itching, seminal emission), constipation, insomnia and disturbed sleep with nightmares, and a range of anxiety disorders!

Names:
Kidney 6, K6, Zhao Hai, Shining Sea or Illuminated Sea.

Where:
This point is located one thumb width below the inside of the anklebone.

How:
Proceed as for acupressure point Spleen 6: sit down and place your left ankle on your right knee. Place your right thumb in the depression right below the ankle bone.
Press with your thumb or knuckle. Increase pressure until you are pressing quite firmly, hold about a minute, and gradually release.
Switch legs and work on the right leg point.

FOOT POINT:

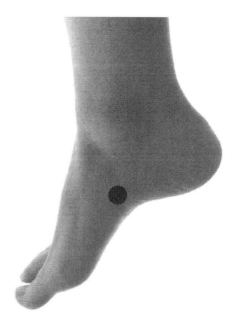

Relieves oedema, especially swollen feet.

Names:
Kidney 2, K2, Ran Gu, Blazing Valley.

Where:
This point is located on the middle of the arch of the foot, midway between the outer tip of the big toe and the back of the heel.

How:
Sit down and place your left ankle on your right knee. Place your right thumb in the depression of the arch. With your thumb perpendicular to the arch, apply firm pressure in the direction of the inner center of the foot.
Press with your thumb or knuckle. Increase pressure until you are pressing quite firmly, hold about a minute, and gradually release.
Switch legs and work on the right foot point.

BALANCE YOUR MOOD SWINGS

Key Acupoints:

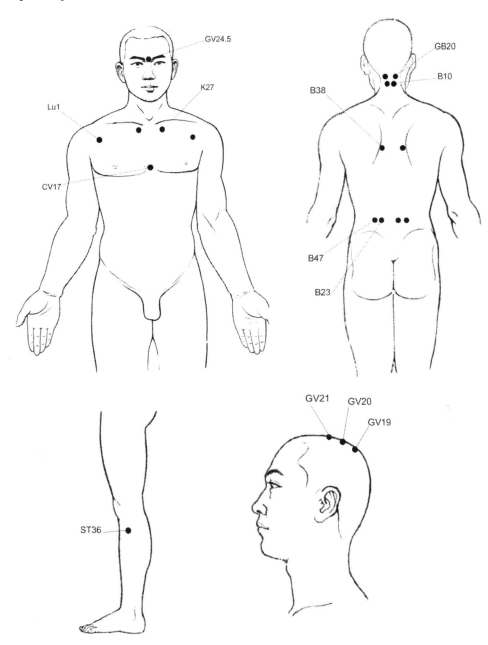

Exercise:

Concentrate on breathing slowly and deeply throughout all of the steps. Deep breathing increases circulation to every part of your body, washes away tension, relieves depression, and infuses your body with vitality.

Lie down on your back:

1. Press B38 (upper back):

Lie down on your back, and place 2 golf or tennis table balls on the floor underneath your upper back between your shoulder blades. If the pressure hurts, cover the balls with a thick towel. Close your eyes, and breathe for 2mn.

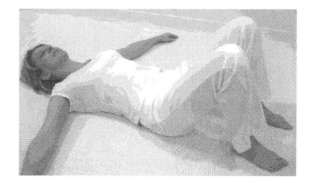
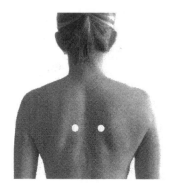

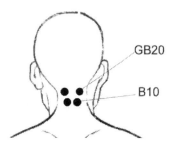

Firmly press B10 and GB20 (neck):

Use your fingertips to firmly press B10 on both sides of the ropy muscles on your neck for 1mn. Then use your thumbs to gradually press up underneath the skull into GB20, as you slowly tilt your head back and breathe deeply for another minute.

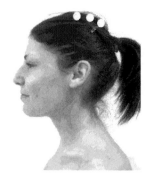

2. Stimulate GV19, GV20 and GV21 (top of the head):

Place your fingertips on the centre on the top of your head, and then briskly rub with all your fingertips to stimulate these 3 antidepressant points for 1mn.

42

3. Firmly press K27 and Lu1 (upper chest):

Use your fingertips on both sides of your chest to firmly press K27 and then Lu1 for 1mn each.

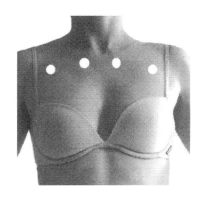

Slowly sit up and continue.

4. Rub B23 and B47 (lower back):

Make fists and place your knuckles against your lower back, 2 inches apart on either side of the spine. Briskly rub your back up and down for 1mn to create heat.

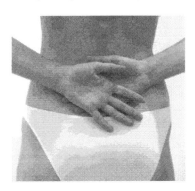 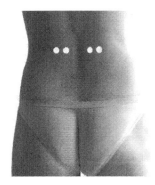

5. Rub St36 (lower leg):

Place your left fist on St36 of your left leg and briskly rub it for 1mn. Then do the same on the other leg.

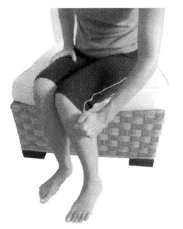 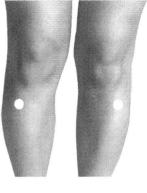

6. Third Eye visualization:

Sitting with your spine straight, eyes closed, chin tilted down slightly, bring your palms together and use your middle and index fingertips to lightly touch the Third Eye point. Take long, slow, deep breaths as you visualize yourself going to a place that makes you feel calm, restful, and safe – a place where you can trust yourself to follow whatever step you need to take to reach fulfillment in your life.

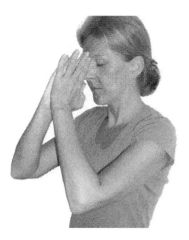
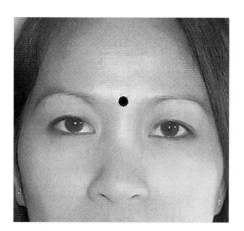

Use all of the fingertips of one hand to gently press the centre of your breastbone as you take several more long, slow, deep breaths to enhance the benefits.

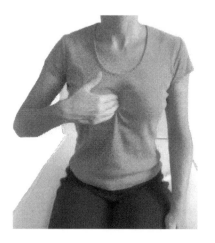
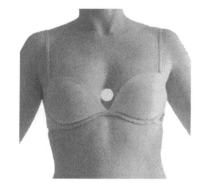

LOWER YOUR ANXIETY

Key Acupoints:

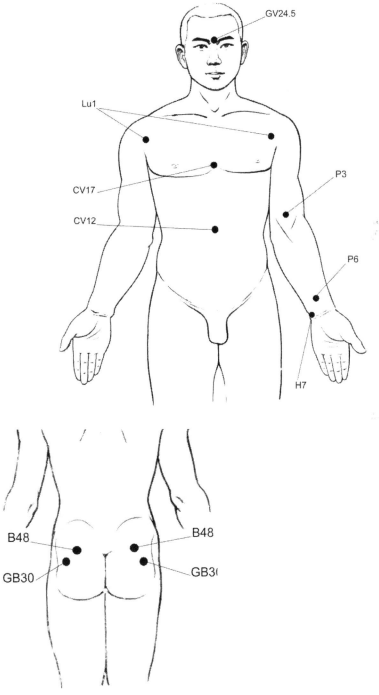

Exercise:

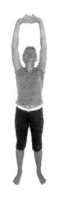

1. Breathe
Stand with your feet comfortably apart and your arms at your sides. Inhale, raising your arms, palms up, out to the sides and then up above your head.

Interlock your fingers, with your palms facing each other. Turn your palms inside out so that your palms face the sky. Inhale, and gently stretch farther upward, with your head tilted back.

Exhale, lowering your chin to your chest and letting your arms float back down to your sides.

Repeat 5 times.

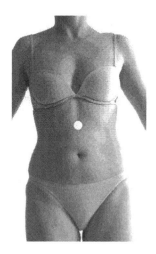

2. Press CV12 (stomach):
Place the fingertips of both hands between your belly button and the base of your breastbone. Gradually apply firm pressure in and upward, leaning your upper body forward, to press deeply into the pit of your stomach, as you breathe deeply for 1mn.

3. Press B48 and GB30 (buttocks):
Place your thumbs on the muscles of your buttocks to press B48 just below your lower back. Take several long, slow, deep breaths as you firmly press inward (toward the centre of your pelvis) for 1mn.

Then make fists and slide them one inch down and one inch outward to press GB30 for another minute.

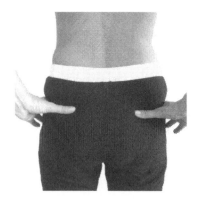
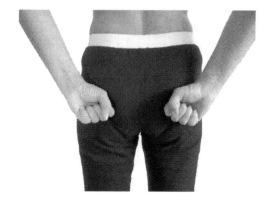

4. Press Lu1 (upper outer chest):

Place your thumbs on the upper, outer portion of your chest, feeling for tension there. Make firm contact with the muscles located 4 finger widths up and 1 finger width inward from your armpit. Close your eyes and concentrate on breathing deeply as you hold those chest points for 1mn.

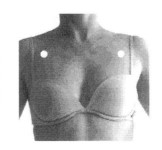

5. Hold P3, press P6 and H7 (inner arm):

Hold P3 with your thumb. Press P6 and H7 with your index and middle fingers for 30 to 60 seconds each. Then switch sides. If you continue to breathe slowly through your nose, you will find that your body is releasing its stress and nervous tension.

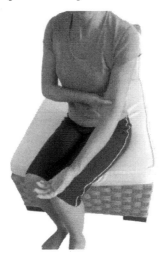
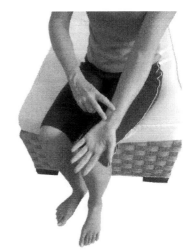

6. Hold GV24.5 with CV17 (face, sternum):

Gently place your right middle fingertip in between your eyebrows on GV24.5 in the slight indentation just above the bridge of the nose. Use the fingertips of your left hand to hold CV17 in the indentations in the centre of your breastbone. Close your eyes and breathe deeply into these points for at least 1mn.

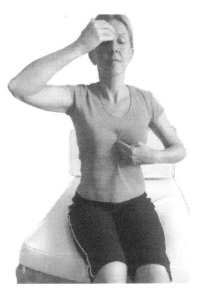

CALM YOUR IRRITABILITY

A Mini-meditation with acupoints

This mini-meditation is for those who find it difficult to meditate, and/or have little time to do it.

Meditation is a powerful source of health and well-being. Even if you do not have enough free time to practice regularly and fully, a few moments of deep breathing while working on specific acupressure points are enough to help you calm down and center.

This mini-meditation takes a few minutes only, and can be practiced anywhere: sitting at your desk, in a taxi, lying on a bed or on a sofa.
It is easy to do, and it stimulates two important acupoints/chakras: the Third Eye (between the eyebrows), and the Hara (below the navel).

In the context of weight management, it is recommended to practice it before eating, to avoid relieving stress with food, and to promote good digestion.

1. Standing up or comfortably seated, close your eyes.

2. Gently put the pulp of your middle finger on the Third Eye (between the eyebrows), and the palm of your other hand on the Hara (between the navel and the pubic bone).

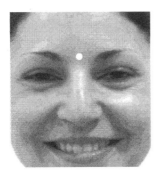 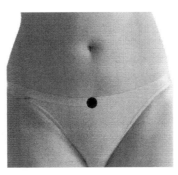 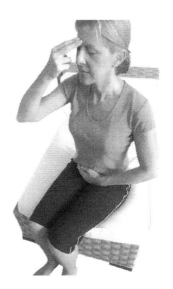

3. Take 5 long... deep.... breaths...

4. Smile, you just gave yourself a beautiful present!

Reduce hot flashes & night sweats

Key Acupoints:

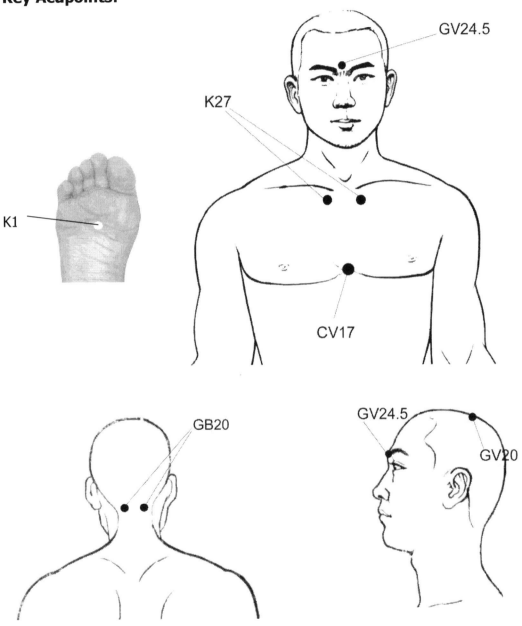

Exercise:

Sit comfortably on a chair.

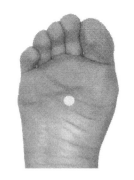

1. Press K1: (foot)
Place your foot on the opposite thigh. Use your thumb to gradually press K1 on the bottom of your left foot. Hold for 1mn and then switch sides.

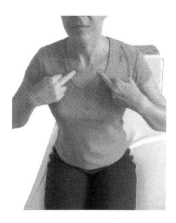

2. Firmly hold both K27 points: (collarbone)
Place your third fingers on both K27. Press firmly as you take slow, deep breaths for 1mn.

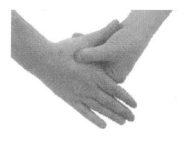

3. Grasp LI4: (hand)
Place our right thumb on the left LI4 point, with your fingertips on the underside below your thumb. Squeeze the thumb and index finger of your right hand together to firmly press into the webbing. Hold for 1mn and then switch sides.

4. Firmly press GB20: (neck)

Place your thumbs underneath the base of your skull, on both GB20. Slowly tilt your head back and breathe deeply. Apply pressure gradually, holding firmly for 1mn as you focus on taking long, slow, deep breaths.

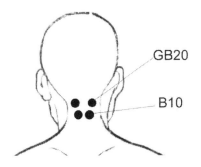

GB20

B10

5. Touch GV20 and GV24.5 (head):

Use the fingertips of your right hand to press GV20. Place the middle fingertip of your left hand lightly on GV24.5 (Third Eye). Focus your attention on that spot with your eyes closed. Straighten your spine and breathe deeply for 2 mn as you hold these nervous system balancing points.

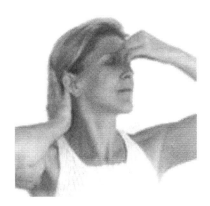

6. Hold CV17 (sternum):

Place all your fingertips on the centre of your breastbone at heart level, fitting them into each indentation. Close your eyes, breathe deeply for 1mn.

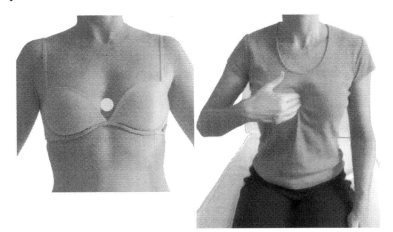

BOOST YOUR ENERGY

The Six Tonic Points

Work on any of these points, anytime, for a few minutes per day.

Sea of Energy (Primal energy)

Names: Conception Vessel 6 (CV6), Sea of Energy, Hara

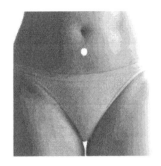

Where: Two finger widths directly below the belly button.
How: You can place your three middle fingers of either hand, on the point area, and press down an inch or two until you reach a firm spot. Or, you can use a more relaxed hold and place the palm of one hand gently on your belly, below your belly button, right over the point. You can use one hand, or both, with one hand over the other. Remember to relax your hands and arms and shoulders. You can hold this while standing (evenly on both feet), sitting (with both feet flat on the ground, back straight), or lying down.
Hold for one or two minutes, while taking slow deep breaths.

Three Miles (Physical energy)

Names: Stomach 36 (St36), Three Miles

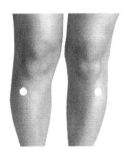

Where: 4 finger widths below the kneecap toward the outside of the shinbone. This point is one of the most difficult to locate.
How: Being in a thick muscular area, it requires strong pressure. There are 2 ways to work this point:

- Sit, legs bent, feet flat on the floor. Press with your thumbs, or roll a small ball on each point. Press as hard as you can.
- Sit, legs stretched on the floor. Lean your body forward to apply a vertical pressure. This technique is more relaxing, and more efficient.

Stimulate this point in the morning, and after lunch (it is located on the Stomach meridian, so you will boost digestion, which uses up to 50% of your vital energy).

Crooked Pond (Psychological energy)
Names: Crooked Pond, Large Intestine 11

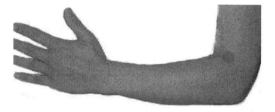

Where: On the top, outer end of the elbow crease. As all acupoints (except the ones on the Conception and the Governor Vessels, which run in the middle line of the body), this point is bilateral: it is located on both arm.

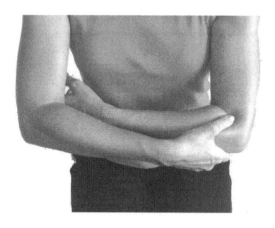

How: Cradle your elbow with your other hand, and use your thumb to hold this point. You can lightly touch it, or massage with a firm touch, in a clockwise motion. Try just one arm, or both, if it's comfortable. Remember to keep your shoulders and arms relaxed.

Elegant Mansion (Tranquility)
Names: Elegant Mansion, Kidneys 27

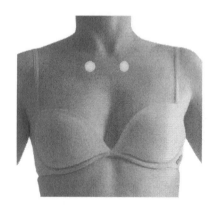

Where: In the hollow below the collarbone next to the breastbone. If you press firmly, these points can be sore.

How: Use the middle finger of both hands, or the thumb and middle finger of one hand. The pressure should be very light. Touch is enough (just place the finger pulp, and do not press). These acupoints are sensitive and reactive. You can feel the pulse just below the skin. Close your eyes, and hold the points for 30 seconds minimum, 1 minute if possible.

Sea of Vitality (Exhaustion)
Names: Bladder 23 and Bladder 47

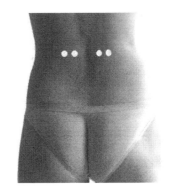

Where: In the lower back, at waist level, between the second and third lumbar vertebrae, 2 to 4 finger widths away from the spine.
B23: 2 finger widths away from the spine.
B47: 4 finger widths away from the spine.

How:
There are 2 ways to work on these points:
- Stand up or sit down: place your hands on your waist, thumbs on the back. Press the points with your thumbs.
- Lie down on your back: place 2 small balls on the floor, at the level of B23 and B47. Let the weight of your body do the pressure work.
  For a softer stimulation, place your hands under your waist, palms on the floor, knuckles up on B23 and B47.

Caution: Do not press on disintegrating discs or fractured or broken bones, If you have a weak back, a few minutes of stationary, light touching instead of pressure can be very healing. See your doctor first if you have any questions or need medical advice.

Bubbling Spring (age-related energy)
Names: Kidney 1, K1, Bubbling Spring

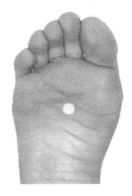

Where: On the centre of the sole of the foot, at the base of the ball of the foot, between the two pads.

How: Sit down on the floor, and
Use your thumb to gradually press on K1. The circular motion technique can also be used.
If you sit on a chair, comfortably place your foot on the opposite lap. You can then reach K1.

Exercise:

Lie down on your back, knees bent, feet flat on the floor.

Place the knuckles of your lose fist on the B47 points in your back (the right fist if the right side of your back is tenser than the left side, the left fist if the left side of your back is tenser).

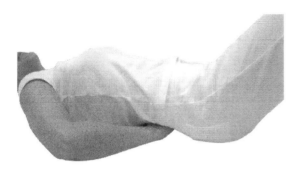 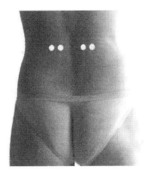

1. With the other hand, **hold B10, K27, CV12 and CV6** in this order for 1mn each. For the double points, hold only the one located on the opposite side of the fist under your back.

B10	K27	CV12

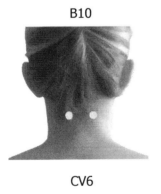 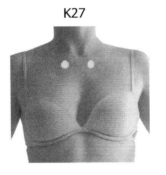 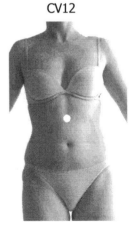

CV6

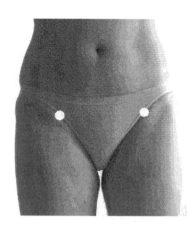

2. Press both Sp13 (pelvic area):

Place all the fingers of both hands on Sp13, located in the middle of the crease where the leg joins the trunk of the body.

3. Firmly press St36 (below the knee):

Keep your legs bent, feet flat on the floor, and sit down. Press your thumbs into St36, four finger widths below the kneecap toward the outside of the shinbone.

SLEEP BETTER

Key Acupoints:

"Joyful Sleep" point:

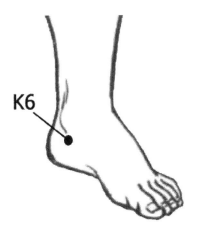

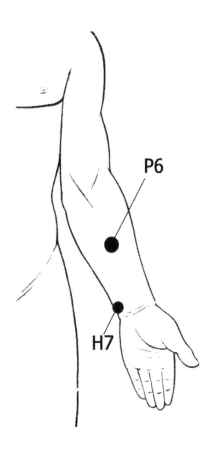

"Calm Sleep" point:

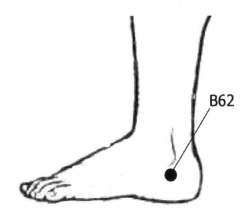

Exercise:

This exercise can be practiced sitting or lying down (even in your bath tub!).

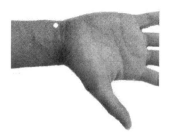

1. Press H7 (wrist crease):
H7 is in the hollow of the wrist crease just below the little finger.
With your right thumb, press on your left H7. Hold for about 1 minute. The pressure should be neutral (not too firm, not too light).
Then switch sides.

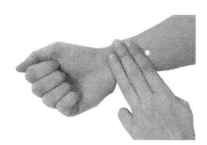

2. Press firmly P6 (inner forearm):
P6 is located on the midline of the forearm, 2 and ½ finger widths below the wrist crease (hence, below the middle finger).
With your right thumb, press firmly on your left P6. Hold for about 1 minute. The pressure should be neutral (not too firm, not too light).
Then switch sides.

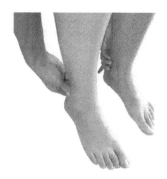

3. Hold both K6 and B62 (ankle):
K6 is in the indentation just below the inner ankle bone, and B62 in the indentation just below the outer ankle bone.
With your feet flat soles on the floor, grab your heels to place your thumbs on your K6 and your middle fingers on your B62.
Hold for 1 minute.

Insomnia during menopause is often due to night sweats and to the irritability generated by estrogens level decrease. Working on the related acupoints should help relieve insomnia too.

If you experience accrued insomnia because of worry, try the exercises described in the "Balance Your Emotions" chapter.

STRENGTHEN YOUR BODY'S RESISTANCE

Key Acupoints:

In addition of the Six Tonic Points, the following acupoints are important points for strengthening the whole body.

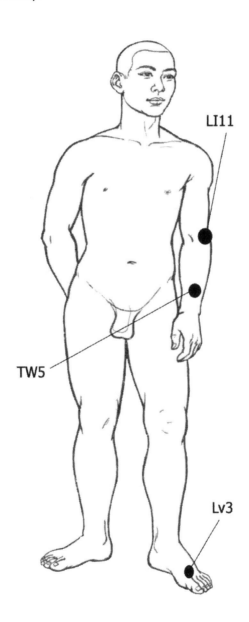

Exercise 1:

Sit down on a comfortable chair.

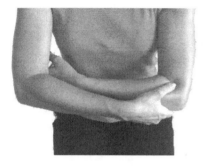

1. Press LI11 (elbow crease):

LI11 is exactly on the outer end of the elbow crease.

Grab your left elbow with your right hand, and place your right thumb on your left LI11. Press for 1 minute. If the point is sore, use the press & release technique.

Then switch sides.

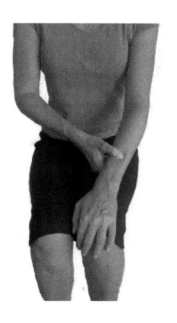

2. Press TW5 (outer forearm):

TW5 is located on the outside forearm, 2 and ½ finger widths above the centre of wrist crease.

Place your left palm on your left lap, so as to extend your forearm and expose its outer side. With your loose right fist, rub TW5 for ½ minute.

Then switch sides.

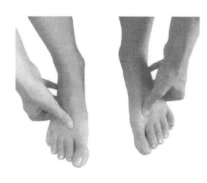

3. Rub Lv3 (top of the foot):

Lv3 is on the top of the foot, in the indentation just between the 1st and 2nd toes bones.

Place your feet flat on the floor. Lift your right foot, and place its heel on your left Lv3. Rub the area for up to 1 minute.

Then switch sides.

Exercise 2: Regulate your vital energy

Lie down on your back, knees bent, feet flat on the floor. Place the middle finger of your left hand on the left B10 point in the back of your neck.

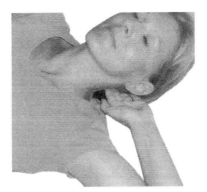 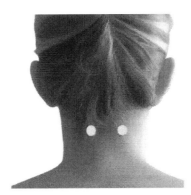

1. With the right hand, **hold St3, and then Sp13** for 1mn each. Hold only the right acupoint.

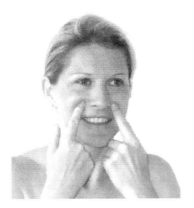 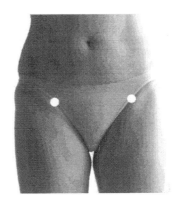

Place your right foot on your left knee

2. Hold at the same time K3 (inner ankle) with your thumb, **and B60 (outer ankle)** with your middle finger for 1mn.

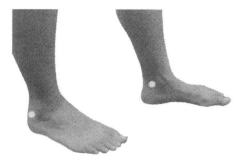

3. With your right hand, hold the toes of your right foot, then left foot.

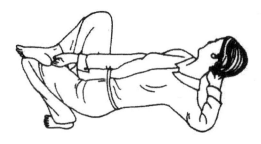

Reconnect with your libido

This complete routine strengthens the sexual energy and the physical energy, and the body sensitivity and sensuality.

Stand up, your feet slightly apart to keep your balance:

1. **Rub B23 and B47 (Sea of Vitality, lower back):**
   With your hands flat, or in a lose fist, rub your lower back up and down and in circular motion for 1 minute. You will feel heat.
   Then grab your waist with your hands, thumbs on the back.
   Press for 1 minute into both B23, located between the spine and the vertical muscle.
   Press for 1 minute into both B47, located 4 finger widths away from the spine.

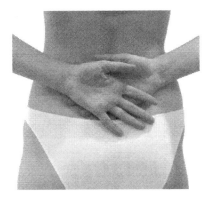 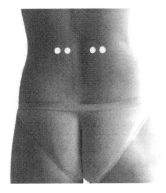

2. **Press CV2 to CV6 (Sea of Energy, abdomen):**
   Place all your fingers along the midline between the navel and the pubic bone. Slightly bend over, to press into CV2 to CV6. Whenever possible during your day, place a hot towel or a bottle of hot water on these points to stimulate them. You can even blow hot air with a hair dryer!

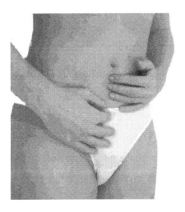

Sit down on the floor:

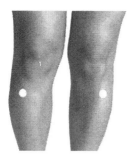 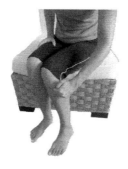

3. Briskly rub St36 (below knee cap).

Stretch your legs in front of you. Place your right heel on your right St36, and rub the point with the heel. You can support your body with your arms if necessary.

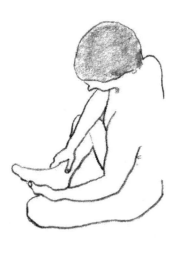 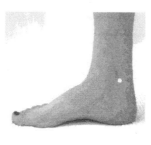 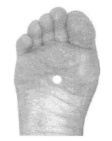

4. Press K1 and K3 (foot sole and inner ankle):

Place your right foot on your left knee. Place your right thumb on K3, located between the ankle bone and the Achilles tendon. Place your left thumb on K1, between the two pads. Breathe deeply while pressing for 1 minute. Then switch sides (left foot on right knee).

Lie down on your stomach:

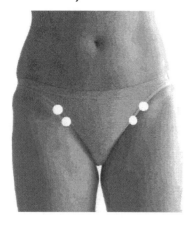

5. Press Sp12 et Sp13 (groin):

Let your forehead rest on the floor. Place your right fist in the crease where the right leg joins the trunk, and your left fist in the crease where the left leg joins the trunk. Join your 2 feet. Inhale while lifting your legs, hold for 30 seconds (breathe!). Exhale while bringing your legs back on the floor. Remove your hands, and relax for 2 minutes.

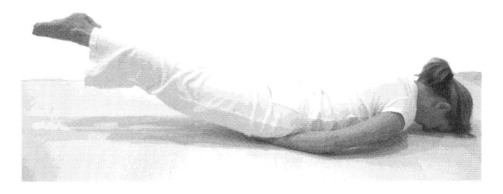

Lie down on your back, bend your knees, place your feet flat on the floor:

6. Press B27 to B34 (Sacral Points, on the sacrum):

The Sacral Points are located along the base of the spine.

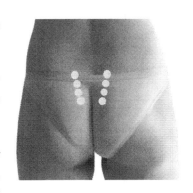

Lift your pelvis, and place your hands under your sacrum one on top of the other, palms facing the floor. Let your pelvis rest on your hands.

Take deep and long breaths, while you slowly sway your legs (together) from right to left and repeat. This movement makes your knuckles press into the Sacral Points, just by using your body weight.

If you prefer, lift your feet, and draw large circles in the air with your knees.

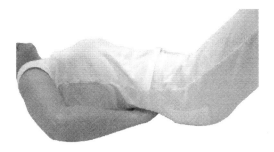

About The Author

Anne Cossé

is a Certified Acupressure Practitioner by the State of California.

She is trained in traditional Shiatsu, Zen Shiatsu, Jin Shin Do, Reflexology, Touch for Health, and Reiki.

She also holds an MBA and a Master of Engineering and has been in the past an Executive in Europe, Asia, and the USA.

Anne has been interviewed by many medias around the world.

Follow her:

www.acupressurewellness.com

www.facialacupressure.com

www.youtube.com/annecosse

www.facebook.com/FacialRejuvenationAcupressure

www.pinterest.com/annecosse

https://plus.google.com/+annecosse

From The Same Author:

The information provided in the "*Embrace Menopause, Natural Relief with Acupressure*" book is for educational and informational purposes only and in no way should be considered as an offering of medical advice. This information should not replace consultation with a competent healthcare professional. The reader should regularly consult a licensed health care professional in matters relating to her menopause and health, and particularly in respect to any symptoms that may require diagnosis or medical attention. The author and publisher are in no way liable for any misuse of the material.

Please note that the author cannot provide personal email consultancy to readers. Thank you for your understanding!

For information: www.acupressurewellness.com

Embrace Menopause, Natural Relief with Acupressure
April 2013
ISBN 979-10-92669-01-5